3 Steps to Wellness

Introduction to basic qigong methods

Jose Beneyto

*For Núria and Irene,
my true treasures*

Download Note

The author declines all responsibility for any injury or accident that may occur to the reader by reading or practicing the material contained in this work.

It is recommended that before following any physical activity you consult an expert in the field and / or medical.

3 Steps to Wellness

Posts by Jose R. Beneyto

Copyright © 2017 Jose Rafael Beneyto Galbis.

Table Of Contents

INTRODUCTION

A person's health is determined by many factors. Some of them are genetic or hereditary. But many others depend on the lifestyle we lead and our habits.

It is in them that we can become more aware and acquire new customs that contribute to improving our health, and therefore our quality of life and well-being.

Traditional Chinese medicine has its own particular way of analyzing a person's health and also establishes a series of factors that influence it.

Some depend on the outside, such as climatic changes and the characteristics of the place where we live.

Others belong to our interior, such as genetics, lifestyle (diet, exercise, rest, etc.) or the control of emotions.

But for centuries they understood that the quality of life of a person could be improved by maintaining a series of habits that had a direct effect on health.

One of the methods they used for this was the practice of a series of exercises that over time became known under the generic name of qìgōng (pronounced "chi kung").

These exercises not only consisted of simple movements, but were accompanied by adequate breathing and concentration. With this they managed to maintain a correct energetic and blood circulation, which they considered key to stay healthy.

But in addition they worked body, energy and mind for an integral care of the human being.

Those primitive exercises were evolving and with time they derived in multitude of different systems depending on the objective that pursued their practitioners.

But in essence they still maintained the circulation of energy and the work of the three aspects as the cornerstone of their practices.

The cultivation of these three aspects (body, energy and mind) is not exclusive to the Chinese tradition.

Throughout history many cultures have understood the composition of the human being and the importance of his work and care.

But it is no less true that within traditional Chinese medicine takes on a special importance and is one of its fundamental basic theories.

For this reason the different systems of qigong and more specifically the Luohan system, become aware of the importance of these three aspects, and develop methods to work and improve them in a harmonious and effective way to improve our welfare.

What I essentially intend to convey is the importance of being aware of the three aspects of which we are made and the three methods that allow us to improve them.

In short, The Three Steps to Wellness.

What I explain in this book is based on the theories and methods that Luohan qigong uses for health care.

But as I explained earlier it is not exclusive to that system and we can find it in most styles of qigong.

THREE TREASURES:
THE KEY TO HEALTH AND WELL-BEING

Within Traditional Chinese Medicine, and especially in the field of qigong, there is a fundamental concept to understand our health, and therefore our well-being and quality of life.

We talk about "The Three Treasures of Health".

In traditional theories they are sometimes described in a somewhat metaphorical and even poetic way.

We have to understand that these theories were developed over centuries in a cultural and social context very different from our own.

Therefore, the way they transmit their knowledge can sometimes be somewhat shocking.

Likewise, the three treasures have been widely studied and used in Chinese medicine and we can find numerous writings that go much deeper into their meaning.

But at the same time, we are talking about a concept that at a basic level is very simple, easy to understand and that will serve as a basis for establishing routines for the care of our health.

For traditional Chinese medicine the human being is basically composed of three things; the physical part, the energy and the mind.

That is to say, we can classify the composition of the human being in three levels; physical, energetic and mental, and each one of them would correspond with each-one of the treasures (jïng 精, qì 氣, shén 神).

1. **The physical part** is everything that we can see and touch.It encompasses our entire physical body, from the skin to the internal organs, passing through bones, muscles, tendons, etc...

This part corresponds to the JING (精), generally translated as essence, and which constitutes the fundamental substances of the human body, being the material base of all its tissues. Therefore, it manifests itself in our physical body.

The robustness of our constitution depends on our jing; a strong jing will manifest in a strong and healthy body. On the contrary, a weak jing will lead to problems of growth, physical weakness, etc.

2. **Energetic part**; it is that which we cannot see, we cannot touch, but which we can feel: in some way it is what gives life and allows our physical part to function. It is what the Chinese call QÌ (pronounced Chi) (氣) (generally translated as "energy").

The qi circulates through a series of channels called JIN-LOU, which allow it to reach all parts of the body. For Chinese medicine there are several types of qi according to their origin, function or location. Various functions are attributed to it, such as propulsion, heating, defense, etc.

3. **Mental part**; it is that which directs the qi (energy) so that the jing (body) can function.

That is, it is our mental activity that will direct the functioning of our body through energy, either consciously or unconsciously. It is what the Chinese call SHÉN (神) (often translated as "spirit", "mind" or "consciousness").

Shen is a very broad and very generic term that refers not only to our mental activity, but also to various external manifestations of our vital activity, such as expression, gaze or general aspect.

Simply put, we are body, mind and energy. Evidently, each of these three aspects can be divided into many sections; the physical body can be divided into systems; there are different types of energy; and the mental aspect can also be divided into conscious, subconscious, and so on.

But the basic idea is that whatever we are made of can be included in one of these three aspects.

An example will help us to better understand the meaning of these three concepts;

Let us focus on one of our arms. That would be the jing, or physical part.   It can be seen and touched.

Now let's move it. For this we need something that we cannot see or touch, but that we can feel: that is the energy, or qi.

And we also need something that gives the order to execute the movement, which is our mind, or shen.

Therefore, we can already see in this example, that these three parts will always go together; my mind (shen) sends energy (qi) to the arm (jing) in order to move it.

Actually, jing, qi and shen are terms that we could analyze and explain in a much more extensive and complete way. But what is really important is to understand that in a very general and very basic way, we are composed of these three aspects.

In this way, if we manage to work and improve each one of them, our health, and therefore our life will be better.

It is important to understand that the three treasures do not function independently.

Our whole body is a unit and we cannot isolate the functioning of one part without influencing the others.

The work on each of them will influence the other two and as a basic rule in most qigong systems, the three treasures must be coordinated to get our practice to give us the desired results.

Today we know that everything in the Universe is energy and emptiness. That is, we live in a vibrational world where everything comes from the same source and manifests in different ways depending on its type or frequency of vibration.

This is consistent with the ancient Chinese concept of qi, which says that this qi energy underlies everything that exists in the universe.

When it condenses it becomes matter and when it is clarified it becomes spirit. Everything lives and vibrates thanks to the qi that flows within it.

From this point of view, the three treasures or three aspects into which we divide the human being are actually different manifestations of the same "life force" or whatever we want to call it. That is why they should always be coordinated and much of our welfare will depend on our body, energy and mind going in the same direction.

Let us then see what methods we will use to achieve this.

THE THREE STEPS TO OUR WELL-BEING

A t this point, and by way of summary, we understand that the human being is composed in a very basic way of three aspects or levels. Although in reality everything is reduced to energy and emptiness, the different vibration of that energy causes it to manifest in three different but interrelated ways; body, energy and mind.

As a consequence, if we work on these three aspects our life will be better, healthier and happier.

Let us see how we will do it;

Mainly we have three methods for the work of the three treasures; movement, breathing and concentration.

— To work the JING, that is to say, our physical part, we are going to use the **movement.**

— For the work of the QI, the energy, we will use the **breath**.

— For the development of SHEN, our mind, we will use **concentration**.

As we saw in the previous chapter, for good health it is important that the three treasures function in a coordinated and unified way. Therefore, their working methods must also be in good health. That is to say, in all our exercises, for them to be really effective, movement must be coordinated with breathing and concentration.

Although there are exercises that emphasize each of the three aspects, the other two will always be present.

As we have already seen, most Chinese qigong systems consider that in order to maintain an optimum state of health it is of vital importance to cultivate the three treasures and maintain a correct energetic circulation throughout the body.

These three methods will allow us to achieve it. They will be our "Three Steps to Wellness".

In the theories of many systems we can see it expressed as "regulating the body, regulating the breath and regulating the mind".

YIN YANG;
THE IMPORTANCE OF BALANCE

Before analyzing in more detail the three tools or steps to work the three treasures, it is very important to know a theory, that of yin and yang. Although it is very widespread and known, it is necessary to clarify its meaning and its application to our organism and well-being, as well as to the exercises we can perform.

Yin (陰) and Yang (陽) is a philosophical concept used in ancient China. It designates a conception of the world, from which Nature and all its functioning are explained.

We can classify all the phenomena that occur in it by means of this theory, and of course, it is also applicable to the human being. Both its anatomy and its actions can be classified according to the concept of yin or yang.

It is also a theory applicable to the exercises of the different qigong systems, and of course, to the method proposed in this book.

Moreover, knowing clearly the concept of yin and yang will be decisive in our work and will help us to achieve one effect or another in our practice. In later chapters we will learn how to apply this knowledge to the exercises and how it influences them.

But first, let us see in a basic but clear way, what is the meaning of this theory.

What is YIN-YANG?

Imagine a hill for a moment. One of its sides is given the sun. On the other side, there is shade.

On the sunny side there is light, heat, and as a consequence there is more activity.

On the shaded side there is cold, dark, and as a consequence there is more stillness.

The sunny part is the yang. The shaded part is the yin.

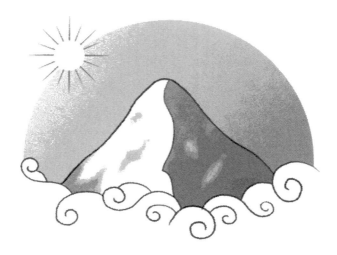

As I explained earlier, this binary conception applies to all aspects of nature.

As a general rule, we can classify anything as yang:

- mobile

- hot

- ascending

- centripetal

- luminous

- outward

- shallow

- business

And we can classify as yin;

- motionless

- chilled

- descending

- centrifugal

- obscure

- inland

- deep

- respite

The human being does not escape this rule. As Su Wen (an ancient Chinese medical book) says: "any tissue structure of the organism can be divided into two opposite parts that are embodied by the yin-yang".

Let's see some examples of this classification;

- Yang: man, part of the body, upper part, surface or exterior, entrails, energy, etc.

- Yin: woman, anterior-medial part of the body, lower part, interior, organs, blood, etc.

Of course, this theory is also applicable to qi gong exercises. Let's take a very general look at examples of how to classify some movements;

- Yang: to inspire, to tense, to ascend, etc.

- Yin; to breathe out, to relax, to go down, etc.

But we must bear in mind that the yin or yang nature of any element or action is not absolute but relative. That is to say, it will be yin or yang in relation to another element.

It is also important to understand that yin and yang are not two different types of energy, but represent the two opposite poles, but at the same time complementary to anything.

This relationship of interdependence between the two elements is perfectly represented by the famous Taiji drawing (supreme essence):

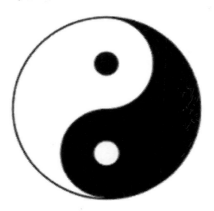

In it we can see represented the main points of this interdependence:

- Yin and yang are opposites. Everything has its opposite, although this is not absolute but relative, since nothing is completely yin or completely yang.

- Yin and yang are interdependent. They cannot exist without each other. As an example, we can be served by day, which cannot exist without night.

- Yin and yang can be further subdivided into yin and yang. Every aspect of yin or yang can in turn be subdivided into yin and yang indefinitely. As an example, the sunny part of a mountain is considered yang. But within it there are things that can be classified momo more yin or yang more.

- Yin and yang consume and generate each other. Yin and yang form a dynamic equilibrium: when one increases, the other decreases. Imbalance is just something circumstantial, because when one grows excessively it forces the other to concentrate, which in the long run causes a new transformation. For example, at dawn, the sun becomes more visible until the darkness completely disappears. When it reaches its maximum brightness, it begins to decrease little by little until it becomes dark again.

- Yin and yang can become their opposites. As in the previous example, day ends up being transformed into night and night into day in a continuous cycle. Another example could be the change of seasons. Cold seasons end in periods of heat and vice versa.

- In yin there is yang and in yang there is yin. Inside yin, there is always something of yang, and on the contrary, inside yang, there remains something of yin. This is represented by small circles of different color.

- Yin and yang are relative. A thing or a natural phenomenon will be yin or yang depending on what you compare it to. For example, water in its liquid state is yin compared to steam, but yang compared to ice.

We can find numerous examples in nature in which these principles of opposition, alternation and transformation are visible;

The dawn supposes an ascent of the energy yang that reaches its maximum at noon. From that moment on, it begins to descend at the same time as the yin energy ascends until it reaches its maximum at midnight. At that moment the yin begins to decrease and the yang grows, repeating the same cycle in which yin and yang are controlled and alternating to maintain a dynamic balance.

It will not be difficult for us to find much more information on the theory of yin and yang. As we have seen, it is applicable to all aspects of life and there are authentic philosophical currents on that theory. But I think that what has been explained so far is enough. I think it is preferable to focus on how we apply that theory to our body, and to our qigong work.

There is one fundamental idea that I think is important to keep;

We can practice qigong exercises in a balanced way, in a yang way, and in a yin way.

Balanced form; the exercises are practiced maintaining the balance between yin and yang obtaining a neutral effect.

Yang form; we will put more emphasis on the phase or on the yang elements of the exercise with the intention of toning, increasing or raising the energy.

Yin form; we will emphasize the phase or yin elements of the exercise with the intention of relaxing, sedating or lowering the energy.

This is a general idea to understand how the theory of yin and yang will help us achieve our goals. There are times when we need to activate, increase our energy. In others we want to relax, eliminate tensions. On the other hand, in others we simply want to work the three treasures in a balanced way.

Although there are exercises designed to achieve one objective or another, small variations in the realization of these will have a different effect.

Later on we will see how we can make a neutral or balanced exercise have a yang or yin effect according to our needs.

STARTING POSITION

Many times people are interested in activities such as qigong and taiji (tai chi) with the intention of learning to relax. Although the truth is that this is not the purpose of these techniques, it is also true that relaxation is a prerequisite for successfully practicing them. We will go a little deeper into this subject later.

Maintaining a good posture is fundamental for this. In fact, learning to place ourselves is the first step in most traditional systems of energetic work.

There is even a well-known practice within the qigong and taiji systems called zhàn zhuāng (literally translated as "standing still like a stake"), which consists of standing still, immobile in a certain position with the aim of improving our posture, eliminating unnecessary tensions, favoring the circulation of qi, calming the mind and a long etcetera.

Here we are not going to tackle that work. We are simply going to see an initial position from which we will start most of the exercises.

At this point we must remember the importance of balance; the theory of yin and yang. All extremes are bad, and an excess of tension can be just as damaging as an excess of relaxation. One of the great objectives of the postures that we are going to learn is to place ourselves in a position as balanced as possible.

Foot Posture

We will stand upright. Feet approximately shoulder width apart. The toes of the feet slightly outward. The knees stretched but not blocked. Pelvic waist in neutral position, with a slight retroversion of the sacrum. The back straight with the look to the front. Arms relaxed, naturally hanging to the sides so that the middle fingers lightly touch the side of the legs.

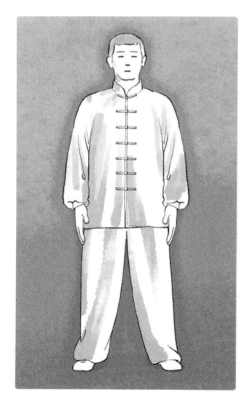

Sitting Position

The sitting posture is a little more Yin than the standing posture. Traditionally it was practiced with the legs crossed and seated on a kind of cushion. But for most people it is more comfortable, and broadly equally effective, to sit in a chair.

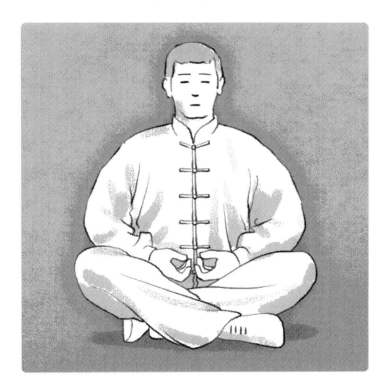

In this variant, you should sit on the edge of the chair without leaning your back against the backrest. Ideally, the knees should be bent 90 degrees so that the thighs are parallel to the floor. They can also be inclined but always with the knees lower than the hips, never the other way around. The feet are still the width of the shoulders, with the tips very slightly outwards or completely parallel. The back is still straight and we keep our eyes on the front. The arms are still naturally relaxed, but now we place them in such a way that the wrists rest on the thighs. At the moment, in a basic position, the palms can be up or down, but always relaxed.

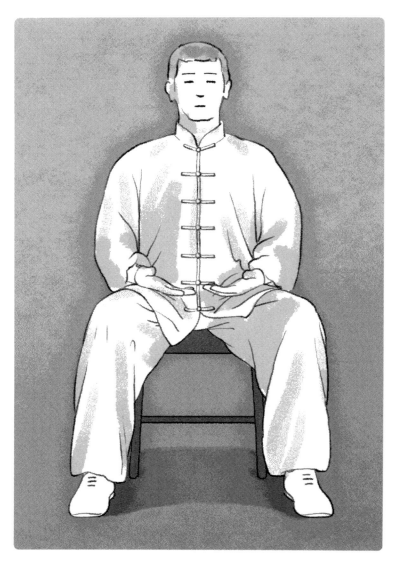

STEP 1 - JING WORK

I n order to really improve our physical body, it is essential to move. In fact, we can use any physical activity that we like and that is healthy. Whether walking, running, dancing or practicing any sport regularly, moderately and preferably aerobically can serve to strengthen our body, our jing.

But the goal sought by qigong goes a little further. Many times we don't only talk about strengthening, but also about regulating or balancing the body. Let us remember that on the one hand we seek to work our jing, but we also want to improve the circulation of energy throughout the body. And movement is an excellent tool to boost blood circulation, and therefore energy, throughout the body. But although any exercise helps that circulation, there are some methods that are more effective and appropriate for it.

In qigong, the balance of the body is usually achieved through a series of stretching and relaxation exercises that help us eliminate excessive tension in the body and provide an optimal state of relaxation.

This relaxation of the body is a prerequisite, along with a proper posture, for blood and energy to circulate freely. This will also allow us to breathe correctly and maintain a balanced mental state.

This type of exercise consists of maneuvers to stretch and relax the different parts of the body, slowly and rhythmically to stimulate circulation.

There are many benefits that we can obtain with the exercises that include such stretching. Apart from stimulating the energetic circulation, different structures or tissues of the body will be benefited;

- ## Muscles;

Being the active part of our locomotor system, they are one of the structures most benefited by stretching.

Stretching helps a correct displacement of the structures that form the muscles, thus ensuring their functionality.

They contribute to maintaining flexibility, adaptability, stability and elasticity, factors that determine the true strength of a muscle.

They help reduce possible contractures, which improves the overall functioning of the muscle.

One of the most interesting effects we get with stretching exercises is drainage; if we compare the muscle with a sponge that in this case is full of blood, when we stretch it we help to empty it, draining the blood that was inside and eliminating toxins and waste products. By relaxing and releasing the stretching, as a sponge would do, the muscle fills again with blood, this time oxygenated, which will receive a greater supply of nutrients. In this way we can promote blood circulation, and therefore energy, in the different muscle groups, improving their nutrition and the elimination of waste products, with all the benefits that this entails.

They help to a correct reciprocal balance between agonist and antagonist.

• Bones and joints;

Stretching stimulates the synovial glands, resulting in increased production of synovial fluid. This benefits all tissues that are nourished by the synovial fluid, especially joint surfaces.

In the stretching phase of most exercises, what we are really looking for is to separate the different bones that make up each joint; that is, to increase the interarticular space for an instant, as indicated in the drawing. This causes a series of compressions-decompressions that also contribute to a better nutrition of the articular cartilages.

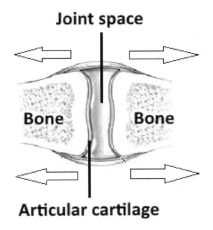

Joint space

Bone　　**Bone**

Articular cartilage

This frees these joints, which helps bone regeneration. This is especially important when it comes to the spinal column, because, even lightly, we help to decompress the space between vertebrae.

In addition, the intra-articular temperature is increased, so that the synovial fluid becomes less viscous and performs its functions better.

It has been shown that moderate physical exercise helps to slow down the loss of bone mass.

By favouring more elastic muscles and without contractures, we manage to eliminate pressures or tensions on the bones, thus avoiding one of the factors that favour bone wear.

• Ligaments;

The separation or decompression of which we spoke previously subjects to certain tension the different ligaments whose function is, precisely, to maintain the joint united. This controlled pressure to which they are subjected helps to strengthen them.

• Tendons;

Another of the great beneficiaries of exercises in this way are the tendons. As I mentioned before, stretching a muscle group actively involves contracting its antagonists. In addition, after a phase of exercise in which we reach its maximum extension we release and contract until it reaches a point at which we start a new stretch. With this what is achieved is that the stretching starts from the contraction of the muscle, turning it in its initial phase into an eccentric stretching. These stretches, since the muscle is still contracted initially, have a special effect on the tendon, which keeps it more elastic and resistant.

In fact, eccentric stretching is an excellent therapeutic weapon in physiotherapy and massage for the treatment of tendon pathologies.

Tendons tend to be one of the most forgotten structures in the work of different physical activities. The practice of qigong helps us fill this gap.

Practice

It is very difficult to teach through a book the correct way to execute the exercises.

What I describe below is just a very basic but very effective example of how with stretching we can improve the circulation of qi, in addition to working and improving our jing.

This is a very popular exercise and is present in some of its versions in most qigong systems.

In the following link (https://youtu.be/oxEzkMD1Oys) you will accede to a video in which you will be able to see its execution. Together with the following instructions you will find it easy to learn.

To start, adopt the first starting position we have seen, the one in which we are standing.

Take a few moments to observe how is your posture, and if it complies with the indications that we gave in the corresponding chapter. Later on, when we have talked about it, you will be able to spend a few minutes regulating your breathing and your mind. For now, it is enough to focus on your posture and remain attentive to the sensations you are feeling.

From here, keeping your arms relaxed, interlace your fingers and place them in front of your abdomen with your palms facing upwards. At the same time, bend your knees slightly. Keep your back straight and look straight ahead. (fig. 1).

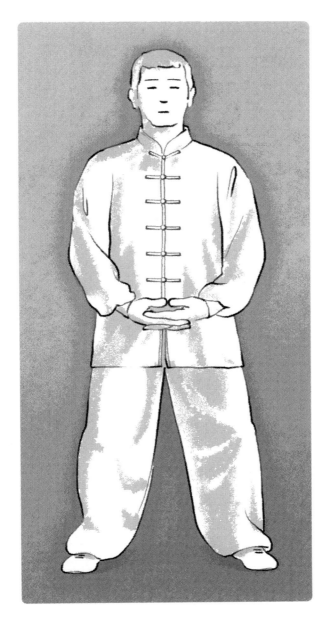

Figure 1

Begin to stretch your legs and at the same time raise your palms in front of your body until your forearms are parallel to the ground. (fig.2)

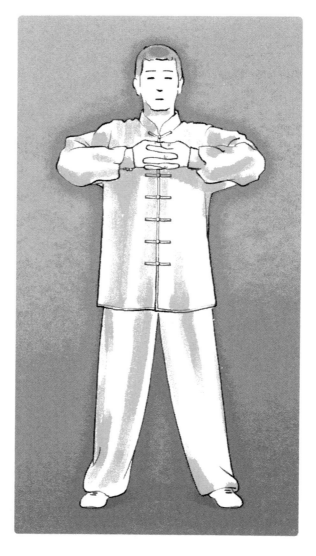

Figure 2

At this point, continue to raise your hands as you turn your palms until they look up again.

Keep going up until your arms are fully stretched. Your legs are stretched, your back straight, and your arms completely stretched with your hands just above your head and your palms facing up (fig.3).

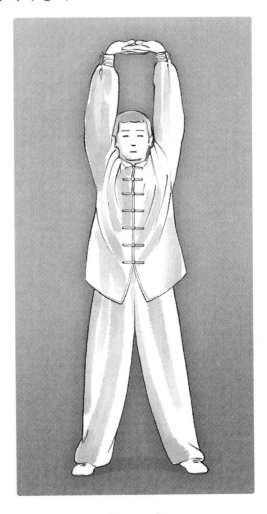

Figure 3

Hold that position for a moment, maintaining the intention (Yi) to keep pushing upwards, even if there is no more movement because it has already reached its maximum extension.

Finally, only if you can maintain your balance, tiptoe yourself with the intention of reaching a little higher. Remember not only to push with your hands, but also with your mind, with your intention. (fig. 4)

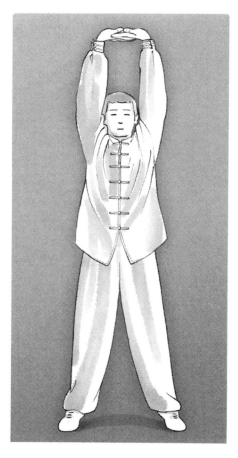

Figure 4

After this, put your feet back on the floor, release your hands, and gently lower your arms sideways until you reach the bottom and return to the starting position (Fig. 5 and 6). Your knees should bend slightly as you lower your arms. Your concentration or mind also relaxes, focusing now on feeling the sensations that relaxation produces after stretching.

We would repeat as many times as we wish.

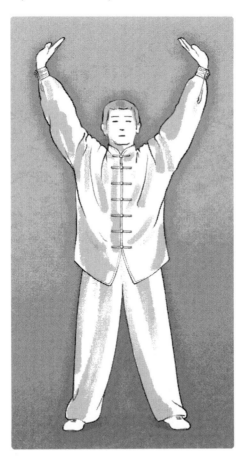

Figure 5

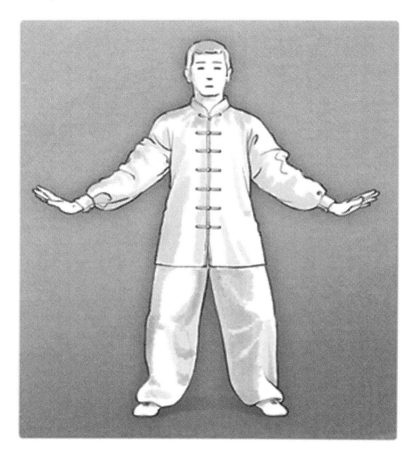

Figure 6

This exercise is mainly intended to stretch the entire musculature of the trunk. This, as we have already seen, will benefit from a greater supply of blood and nutrients.

But we also subject the internal organs to a kind of pressure-decompression, producing a pumping effect, which will also benefit from a better blood supply and energy.

No less important is the stretching on the spinal column, seeking to decompress for a few moments the vertebrae, thus helping to improve the state of the different structures that accompany them (discs, ligaments, etc.).

We also stretch part of the muscles of the legs and arms.

Its practice helps us to feel more awake, but at the same time more relaxed. At first it is better not to think about breathing, but we will see how the body naturally breathes in when you stretch your arms, and releases the air when you relax and bend them.

Keep your eyes in front of you throughout the exercise. It will help to be upright and maintain balance when tiptoeing. Don't be in a hurry to do it and be attentive to the sensations that are produced. Remember the importance of balance, avoiding an excess of tension when stretching and an excess of relaxation when releasing.

Do several repetitions, and you will realize that you somehow remember the cycle of the day or seasons, respecting the theory of yin and yang. From the relaxation of the beginning of the movement (yin) it begins to rise and stretch until reaching its maximum extension (yang), and from there it decreases again and reaches the low to start the cycle again.

STEP 2 - QI WORK

For the specific work of the qi aspect, we are going to use breathing. Although, as we can see, movement and concentration also help to mobilize energy and carry it wherever we want, in our system the work of different types of breathing to achieve this task is especially important.

According to traditional Chinese medicine, breathing drives the movement of qi throughout the body. Only by breathing are we able to accelerate or slow down our heart rate (by making shorter or longer breaths). As a consequence we can understand that with breathing we can influence the circulation of blood, and therefore, of energy.

To work on our breathing is to become aware of it and to control it. Our usual way of breathing is constantly affected by factors such as conversation, emotional factors, bad postures or simply by stress and fatigue, making it most of the time too superficial.

Since breathing is in charge of boosting energy, an erratic, distracted and superficial way of breathing will negatively affect the energetic circulation through our organism.

Therefore, to balance and facilitate the movement of energy (and with it the blood with all its nutrients) through our body is essential to take control and balance breathing.

Let's look at some of the general benefits that breathing exercises can bring us;

Within the theories of traditional Chinese medicine, it is considered that breathing drives the movement of qi. In this way, improving our breathing will contribute to promote the circulation of energy, and as a consequence of blood, throughout our body.

They produce an increase in the elasticity of the lungs, and therefore their breathing capacity. This benefit is maintained throughout the day and not only during the practice of the exercises.

It improves the oxygenation of the whole body and its tissues, contributing in this way to improve the functioning of its different systems. This provokes a better feeding of these tissues and helps the elimination of waste.

Through the movements of the different muscles that we will use to breathe, especially the diaphragm, the internal organs receive a massage. This will stimulate blood circulation through these organs (kidneys, liver, spleen, heart ...).

Breathing exercises will help us to achieve a state of greater relaxation and mental calm. But at the same time we can also contribute to a greater state of alertness and mental clarity.

Breathing exercises will not only help us to bring energy to different points or areas, but we can also obtain various effects on it such as speeding up or slowing down its circulation.

Therefore, there are many different types of breathing in qigong, which we will use depending on the effect we want to achieve.

Two Basic Ways Of Breathing

One of the main objectives with which we will practice it will be to help us direct the energy to different areas.

Basically there are two types of breathing that will help us to mobilize the energy in a concrete way.   That is to say, with them we will influence the movement of the qi and the zones where we are going to direct it.

Let's see what these two types of breathing are;

a) Natural or linear breathing

b) Breathing for heights or zones

A. -Natural Or Linear Breathing

In this type of breathing we simply breathe in through the nose and breathe out through the mouth. That's why we call it natural breathing. We also call it linear breathing because this is the effect we get at the energetic level; when we breathe in energy goes up, and when we breathe out energy goes down, in a linear way.

It is a basic type of breathing on which we can begin to work.

The first step is for the practitioner to be aware of the breath. First without any movement, and then with the different exercises, we must learn to feel our breathing rhythm. Little by little we will try to make the breathing deeper but never without forcing it.

Here we will begin to train what I call the "concept of the bottle"; we will imagine that our trunk (actually our lungs) are like a bottle that we are going to fill. If we put that bottle in the tap, it will fill from the bottom up and when we turn it over to empty it, again it will be the bottom of the bottle that will be emptied first. When we fill our lungs with air (which will be reflected in the movement of our body), they will begin to fill from the bottom up, and when exhaling, as the example of the bottle, the lower part will be the first to empty.

Once we manage to breathe deeply, paused, controlled and in the way we have just seen, we will start to incorporate different types of breathing. This is, for example, yang type breathing, yin type, retention, etc. Later I will delve into all those breathing methods.

B. Breathing For Heights Or Zones

The most common is to breathe automatically and involuntarily without paying attention to this process.

But we can also take control and we will realize that to breathe we need the action of different muscles.

Depending on the musculature that we use the air will be directed to different areas of the lungs, thus producing various effects on our body. Within many qigong systems, three different types of breathing are usually differentiated according to the musculature that we use and therefore the area of the lungs where the air will be directed:

- **LOW ZONE:** often referred to as diaphragmatic or abdominal breathing. It is regulated by the movement of the diaphragm. When inspired, it moves downward, thus reaching the air to the deepest part of the lungs. This causes the abdominal organs to move downward and outward on inspiration, and return to their place on expiration. This produces a movement of pumping or massage, and with this we achieve a greater circulation of blood and therefore energy throughout the lower area of our body. Using terms of Chinese medicine, we can say that we are working the **lower jiāo**. All this will help to improve all the tissues located in this area, especially the corresponding internal organs.

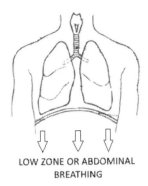

LOW ZONE OR ABDOMINAL
BREATHING

- **MEDIUM ZONE:** also known as thoracic or intercostal breathing. It depends on the intercostal muscles, which are located between the ribs. During inspiration these muscles expand, pushing the ribs outwards and widening the rib cage. During exhalation they return to their initial state.   With this we help blood and energy circulate throughout the middle area of our body, which in Chinese medicine is known as **jiāo medium**. As a consequence, all the tissues of the middle zone will benefit, especially the internal organs included in it.

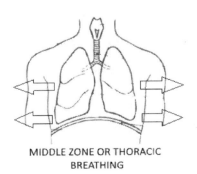

MIDDLE ZONE OR THORACIC
BREATHING

- **HIGH ZONE:** sometimes known as clavicular respiration. On this occasion it is the clavicles that when breathing in rise to open the upper part of the lungs, getting the air to go to that area. During exhalation they relax and return to their initial position. Therefore, it will be the entire upper zone, and especially the corresponding internal organs, that will benefit from the pumping or massage produced by breathing. In terms of Chinese medicine we will say that we are working the **upper jiāo**

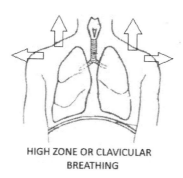

HIGH ZONE OR CLAVICULAR
BREATHING

In short, what we seek to bring the air to each of the heights we have seen. With this we achieve that the muscles in charge of directing the air to each one of them contract and relax, which produces a pressure and relaxation on the organic structures located in each one of the heights.

This produces an effect similar to the one we obtain with a massage; to activate the circulation of the blood and of the energy to each one of those heights. This will improve the functioning and therefore the health of the whole area, especially the corresponding internal organs. This is due to the greater blood supply, which will contribute to better nutrition of all tissues and better waste disposal.

Six Breathing Systems

As we have just seen, the two basic methods of breathing serve to direct the movement of the qi and the areas where we want to work.

But with the breathing we can achieve different effects on the energy independently of the zone that we are working.

Although many times we are not conscious, the respiratory cycle consists of four distinct phases: inspiration, pause, exhalation, pause.

By varying the duration and/or intensity of each of them we will be able to achieve different effects on our organism.

Traditionally, in the Luohan qigong six systems or methods of breathing are taught with their corresponding objectives.

Let's see which are these six breathing systems;

1. Balanced breathing (neutral)

2. Yang type breathing

3. Yin type breathing

4. Explosion breathing (pao sik)

5. Turtle breathing (quai sik)

6. Embryonic breathing (reverse)

BUT FIRST...BREATHE THROUGH THE NOSE OR THROUGH THE MOUTH?

Once again, it depends on what we want to achieve. The nose is specifically designed for breathing, and is responsible for filtering and heating the air.

But breathing through the mouth allows us to get more air in and out.

As a general rule, you breathe in and out through your nose when you want to keep the energy inside more and when the Qi movement you are looking for is less.

It is also advisable when the temperature is very cold and we need to heat the air. From an energetic point of view, inhaling and exhaling through the nose has a more invigorating effect on qi.

When we breathe in through the nose and exhale through the mouth, we tend to get a greater movement of qi, as the air can come out more freely through the mouth. As a general rule, in this variant, when inhaling through the nose we raise the qi, and when exhaling through the mouth we lower the qi.

We can also inspire through the mouth. Although it is not the most advisable form for daily life there are occasions in which we can use it. Especially when we need a bigger air intake. When we find ourselves in situations, such as, for example, after a strenuous effort, the body will take air through the mouth in a natural way because it allows greater entry of this and therefore greater supply of oxygen.

In more advanced works of Luohan qigong, one breathes through the mouth to direct the air to concrete zones or areas.

It is interesting to note that there are devices for the recovery of patients with various ailments in which they must blow with the intention of moving a series of balls that are inside. This device is used to strengthen and increase lung capacity and in these exercises is inspired and exhaled through the mouth. This gives us to understand that although it is not the most adequate way to breathe during the day to day, in concrete situations it is perfectly valid to use the mouth to breathe.

Now yes, let's look at the six types of breathing;

Balanced Breathing

Starting from the fact that we already have clear concepts of Yin and Yang, we will define balanced breathing as that which has a neutral effect on our organism.

That is to say, with it we do not intend to activate ourselves (yang) nor sedate ourselves (yin), what we are looking for is a neutral or equilibrium effect. We will seek to promote the circulation of energy, but in a balanced way.

To achieve this we will focus on our inspiration lasting the same as our exhalation. Generally, and as a reference, we will count to three when we breathe in and we will also count to three when we breathe out. Obviously this count of three will be faster or slower depending on each person's lung capacity. It is simply a matter of counting to make inspiration and exhalation last the same.

Balanced breathing is a basic method that will help us focus, relax and become aware of our body as well as eliminate tensions and promote proper circulation of qi.

We must bear in mind that you should never force your breath. Normally it is advised not to fill our lungs by inhaling more than 70 percent of their capacity. This will avoid unnecessary tensions and a greater use of the inspired air.

Try to take an inspiration by filling the whole of your lungs. You will soon notice that you are over-tensioned and forced to let go of the air quickly, losing control of the exhalation.

Our intention is to become aware of the breath and learn to control it and "play" with the four phases that compose it in order to obtain different answers.

If instead of filling the lungs completely, we do it approximately 70 percent, we will realize that we can retain the air much longer if we want and then we can control the expiration much better and make it longer, shorter, intense or soft according to our will.

Practice

Adopt one of the two starting positions that we have seen. You can stand, or sit, whichever is most comfortable for you.

Allow yourself a few seconds, or as much time as you consider necessary, to focus on your position, analysing the points we saw; feet shoulder width apart, back straight, arms relaxed and gaze forward. You can keep your eyes open, but I advise you to close them slightly, it will help you isolate yourself from the outside and focus on yourself.

Once you have regulated your body, we focus on your breathing. For now, breathe in through your nose and breathe out through your nose or through your nose, whichever is most comfortable for you. Feel your breath and be aware of its four phases that are happening cyclically. Little by little, make your breathing deeper, longer, softer and rhythmic, avoiding filling your lungs too much and controlling that when you breathe out, you don't blow all the air out.

Don't worry if at first you get distracted or your thoughts take you somewhere else. When you realize it, simply focus on your breathing again.

After a while, which can be several minutes or with the practice of just a few breaths, we will become aware of the duration of our breathing. Let's try to make the inspiration and the exhalation last the same. As a guide you can count up to three when you breathe in and also up to three when you breathe out.

With this we will get a neutral effect on the qi. We simply manage to make it circulate (in addition to all the benefits we saw the breathing exercises can bring us), but in a more neutral way.

Yang Breathing

In this type of breathing we will make the inspiration longer than the exhalation. A similar effect would also be achieved by placing more emphasis on inspiration (making it stronger).

To achieve our goal, we would count to four when inhaling and up to three when exhaling.

The effect we get with this type of breathing is a yang job; raising energy, stretching our body, accelerating circulation, etc.

Practice

As with the previous exercise, choose the starting position that is most comfortable for you. Allow yourself a little time to focus and regulate your breathing. After a few repetitions, focus on the times and make the inspiration a little longer than the exhalation. As indicated, a good guide can be to count up to four in the inspiration and up to three in the exhalation.

With it we will obtain a more toning effect, more yang; it will help us to activate ourselves, to increase our energy, to revitalize ourselves, etc.

Yin Breathing

With this type of breathing we get the opposite effect, ie get a yin work, lower the energy, relax the body, sedate the circulation, etc..

In order to achieve this we will make the inspiration shorter than the exhalation. On this occasion it would also be worth putting more emphasis on exhalation (making it stronger or more pronounced).

Returning to the beads, we'll count to three when breathing in and up to four when breathing out.

Practice

Exactly the same as the previous ones, after adopting a starting, regular posture and paying attention to our breathing, we will focus on the times, counting now up to three when inhaling and up to four when exhaling.

This gives us a more relaxing, calming and sedative effect. In other words, a more yin effect.

Only with this type of basic breathing and understanding the theory of yin and yang, we have already seen how we can obtain different effects in our body by making small variations in the duration of the different phases of breathing.

It is something basic, simple, but extremely useful for our practice. What we have just seen is applicable to most exercises, and understanding it correctly, we can adapt them to our objectives, depending on whether we seek to work in a more active, stimulating, more relaxing, softer or simply want to do a more balanced work.

On occasions when we need a plus of vitality (tiredness, apathy, etc.), practicing yang type breathing can help us.

On the contrary, in situations where we need to relax (stress, tension, worry, etc.) breathing in a yin way can help us.

If we simply want to mobilize energy, focus the mind and benefit our overall health and well-being, balanced breathing will be adequate.

There is another way to transform our neutral breathing into yang or yin:

Faster breathing will force us to do a more shallow breathing, which will get a yang effect, helping to raise our pulsations, our energy, etc. On the contrary, a slower breathing will lead us to make it deeper, which will get a more Yin effect, more relaxation, lower our heart rate, etc..

Quai Sik (Turtle Breathing)

As we have already seen, the respiratory cycle is composed of four phases;

Inspiration-pause-expiration-pause

Previously we have seen how we can vary the duration of inspiration and expiration according to our needs.

But we can also use the existing pauses between the two to achieve certain objectives.

The so-called "quai sik" or breathing of the turtle consists of holding the breath. That is, we increase the duration of some of these breaks with a specific purpose.

In a very general way, we can say that within the Luohan qigong we use this type of breathing with the intention of maintaining the qi or energy in a specific area during a certain time. The duration of retention that we practice in our system is usually quite short, usually one or two seconds. It is usually done together with a pause in the movement of the exercise that we are doing and concentrating on the area or point where we want to keep the energy.

There are two variants of this type of breathing; the one in which we pause after inspiration and the one we do after we exhale. Let's see a little more detail each one of them.

1- It consists of inspiring, keeping the air and then releasing it. It has a more yang effect, that is, we seek to tone up the point or area that we are working on.

2- This time we exhale, then we pause, then continue with inspiration. On this occasion it has a more yin effect. We seek to hold the qi in a specific area or point but with a more relaxing purpose.

Practice

Adopt a starting position. Take a few moments to become aware of your breathing. When you feel ready, inspire and hold for a few seconds. At the beginning, one or two seconds is enough. Never exceed three. Do not make longer retentions without the supervision of a professional.

There are many benefits that this small retention gives us. But at the energy level in qigong it serves as an invigorating, accumulator of qi. One of my teachers used to say that he used it to "build qi".

Then continue with a few balanced breaths. After a few repetitions, take a short pause after expiration. They serve the same recommendations as before. Between 1-3 seconds is more than enough. You will notice that the effect you get now is more relaxing, more Yin.

Pao Sik (Breathing With Explosion)

This type of breathing consists of releasing the air suddenly after inspiration. It is usually used with the aim of eliminating tension and promoting the circulation of qi. It favours relaxation and the unblocking of the energetic and blood circulation.

It is therefore very useful in situations of worry, stress, stiffness and muscular and mental tension.

Very often it is combined with the quai sik or turtle breathing. In other words, after inspiration we would hold our breath for a few seconds and then suddenly release the air.

With this combination we manage to take the energy to a certain area to then obtain a relaxation effect and get that energy can circulate properly. We manage to tone the qi at the same time that we manage to relax the musculature.

Again we have two ways of doing this type of breathing;

The first variant consists of expelling all the air that we have inspired previously. With this we get a greater feeling of unblocking but has the disadvantage that if practiced several times leads to an excessive loss of qi.

The second way we have to practice it is to release just a little bit of air after inspiration and then continue with a normal exhalation, ie softer and more controlled.

It is the most used form of the two, as it allows to relax an area without loss of qi

Practice

Choose a starting posture. Take some time to focus and regulate your breathing. Now I advise you to breathe in through your nose and breathe out through your mouth. After a few repetitions, breathe in, make a brief air retention and then release a part of the blow and continue exhaling as much air as you have left. It may emit a sound when you release part of the air with a blow. This is normal.

You will notice a revitalizing effect as well as a relaxing one. It will help to release tension.

Embryonic Breathing (Reverse)

By reverse breathing we mean that which, unlike normal breathing, when we breathe in we contract the abdomen by moving all its walls inwards. During exhalation these walls expand towards the outside as if we were relaxing them.

This results in greater pressure on the internal organs, since to the pressure exerted by the diaphragm downwards when inhaling, we add the pressure exerted by the abdominal walls inwards. Therefore, we are able to increase the massage and pumping effect that these muscles exert on all internal organs during breathing.

In our system it is also known as embryonic breathing because we usually put our mind or concentration on the navel during its realization. In this way we are able to work especially on the jing (essence).

Practice

Take a starting position. Now join your palms together and place them above your navel. Take a few natural, balanced breaths. You will notice that breathing in expands the abdomen and breathing out contracts.

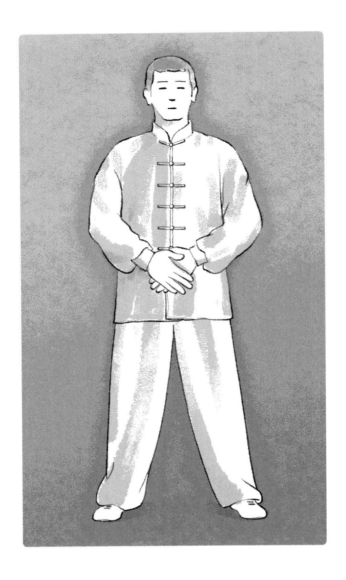

Try to reverse the process; breathe in, but don't allow the abdomen to expand, and consciously push it a little inward. As you release the air relax and allow it to expand now. At first it may seem a little strange and it may cost you, but over time it will come out more naturally.

Personally, I like to do this type of exhalation through the nose, both when inhaling and when exhaling.

You will notice a greater compression of the abdomen as you breathe in and a greater release as you release the air. This allows you to condense the qi more, i.e. attract it more towards the lower abdomen. It also increases the pressure exerted on the internal organs.

We have already seen the two basic types and the six methods of breathing.

We can apply any of the six methods to the two basic forms we have seen of breathing.

That is, we can make a natural or linear breath neutral, yang type or yin type. We can also add quai sik, pao sik and even make it embryonic.

We can do the same with each of the heights.

The possibilities are enormous, but with time and practice we can understand that there are combinations that are much more logical and are the ones that usually appear in the different exercises of qigong.

STEP 3 - SHEN WORK

As we saw earlier, shen is actually a very broad concept that goes beyond what we Westerners understand by "mind". When we speak of shen, apart from the mental activity itself, we also refer to the different expressions of a person's vitality; look, way of speaking, etc.

For the work of our shen, we will use concentration. More concretely, we will work on a Chinese concept called "YI", which means "intention".

In ancient qigong theories it is often said that "wherever the mind is, there the qi will be". This is the fundamental and most important idea about shen training.

Therefore, our intention will be to learn to direct our mind to the places where we want to direct our energy.

We also know that what we think about expands. In other words, we attract what we think. Therefore, a relaxed, positive and focused attitude on what we are working on will help to circulate the qi correctly.

Somehow, what we want to achieve with most qigong exercises is full attention to what we are doing. Our mind or intention, i.e. our YI, must be coordinated with movement and breathing at all times.

A yi focused on the present, on what we are doing in each moment, in harmony with movement and breathing, will help us to have a healthier shen (mind).

In some Eastern traditions the mind is compared to a playful and mischievous monkey. Such a monkey is always moving and doing mischief. We can't make it sit still, as it would go against its nature. But we can give him a toy so that he can entertain himself and forget his mischiefs. Following this analogy, our mind (monkey) is always full of ideas and thoughts (mischief). We cannot empty it of ideas but we can make it focus on something concrete (toy) so that it forgets other thoughts. For example, focusing for a while on our breathing would help us to forget other thoughts, as we would keep it ¨entretenida¨.

Somehow, it's about taking control of where we want our thoughts to go. In our case, the mind, or more exactly our intention, must be coordinated with our movement and our breathing to bring the qi to the area of the body we are working on.

In this way, we continue with the idea that the three treasures, jing, qi and shen must always be coordinated.

Practice

As you have seen, the work of our mind, or more exactly of our intention or YI, is present continuously. It is in everything we do. But let's see an example of how we can use our mind to take qi to certain places.

For this we are going to adopt a starting position. Although any of the two we know are worth it, I recommend that you choose the sitting position. You do not need to sit on a cushion with your legs crossed. Sitting correctly on a chair is more than enough.

Our intention will be to take the qi to three points or areas that in Chinese medicine are considered very important and you can see in the picture. You do not need to know the function of these points. But for your information, I will briefly describe what this is about;

The three dāntián are three zones located in the anterior part of the body, a little towards the interior. They are not specific points, but slightly wider areas. The Chinese concept of dāntián "(丹田)" consists of two parts;

- dān (丹); refers to a certain substance or elixir that was supposed to provide health and longevity.

SĀN DĀNTIÁN
三丹田

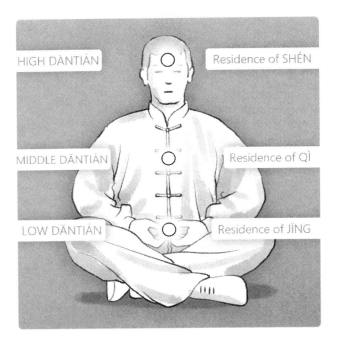

HIGH DĀNTIÁN   Residence of SHÉN

MIDDLE DĀNTIÁN   Residence of QÌ

LOW DĀNTIÁN   Residence of JĪNG

Let's start with the first of them; we already have the right position and we have regulated our breathing.

Now, before starting a new inspiration, we place our mind, our intention, in the superior dantian. It is as if with the mind we tell the qi where we want it to go. Afterwards we continue to inspire, keeping our intention in that area. After a brief pause, we exhale and relax our mind at the same time as the air comes out. We would repeat the process three or four times in each of the zones; in each of the three dantian.

This is just one example of how we use intention to direct the qi. It would actually serve any point or area of the body. Wherever we pay attention, the qi will go.

The important thing is to understand that the mind must always be coordinated with movement and breathing.

When we stretch, we must accompany our intention, increasing the sensation of stretching.

When breathing, the mind also accompanies and concentrates on each of the four phases.

ABOUT RELAXATION

One of the questions that most often attracts people who come to qigong and taiji classes is relaxation.

My answer is always the same; the goal of qigong and taiji is not to relax. But it is also true that relaxation is a prerequisite for practicing these disciplines correctly.

As it could not be otherwise, from our perspective relaxation is valued in relation to the three treasures.

The main objective of qigong exercises is to achieve a correct circulation of qi throughout the body. For this, it is essential to be relaxed. We consider that relaxation has several levels, and as you can imagine, they correspond to the three treasures.   The body, the breath, and the mind must be relaxed.

A body that is not well placed (posture) will not be able, or at least it will be very difficult, to relax. For a body that is not relaxed can not flow the qi correctly. But neither can it do it without a fluid, rhythmic and deep breathing (regardless of whether we work it yin, yang or neutral). And finally, without a serene and balanced mind we will not achieve it either.

As you can already imagine at this point, we seek to find that relaxation from movement, from breathing and from intention, those three steps that can lead us towards our well-being.

It is a broad topic that undoubtedly gives for another book that explains in much more detail how to reach that state of relaxation.

But as always, we must avoid extremes and respect the rule of yin and yang. An excess of tension can be just as bad as an excess of relaxation. As another one of my teachers used to explain; "you have to be relaxed, but not soft. You always have to maintain a certain vital tone.

As we saw in the corresponding chapter, the stretching (the one explained in this book is an excellent example) practiced in the different qigong systems helps to relax the different body structures, especially the muscles, which are its active part.

Deep, paused and conscious breathing not only mobilizes the circulation of energy and blood, but also helps to eliminate tension and thus promote a state of relaxation. We already saw that yin-type breathing, holding the air and then releasing it all at once, etc. could help us to do this.

Finally, using the intention in the different exercises and focusing on what we are doing in each moment helps us to forget about other issues or thoughts that may generate tension or worry, thus allowing us to remain more relaxed.

In short, the practice of qigong exercises, or in other words, of the three steps towards our well-being that we have already analysed, imply an intrinsic work of relaxation.

CONCLUSION

The different existing systems of qigong are the heritage of many generations of practitioners who have been perfecting their theories and practices to achieve their goals.

There are very simple methods and others really extensive and complex. Many of them are based on medical theories that must be known to reach their highest levels.

It usually requires the guidance of a qualified teacher and some time of practice depending on the system being practiced. It is really difficult, very probably impossible, to transmit this knowledge through a book. Definitely impossible if you want to learn exclusively from a book.

But it is equally true that it is not necessary to learn the totality of a qigong system or to be a great expert to obtain some of its benefits.

The intention of this book is to analyze in a very basic and simple way the methods used by most qigong systems and the benefits they can bring us.

I especially rely on the knowledge my teachers have given me about the style I practice. Further information on this system can be found in my previous book "Lohan Chi kung. Treasure for Health" (amzn.to/2ao9Iqx). In it, I make an introduction to the different categories of qigong. I explain the history of Luohan gong, its objectives and working methods. I also show the essential points for its practice.

The methods I explain in this book are mainly based on that system.

To become aware that we are body, energy and mind and that we can work with movement, breathing and concentration. To know that they are three indivisible aspects and must be coordinated. Knowing simple exercises that can help us improve them can be a good starting point to improve our welfare.

Thank you!

I really hope that you liked this little book and that it will be useful. If so, I would be very happy if you rate Amazon positively.

Your opinion is very important, and not only helps to position the book among the many that exist, but is a recognition of the effort and work involved in writing it.

Anyway, thank you for buying it and devoting your time to its reading. Thank you and see you soon!

ABOUT THE AUTHOR

Jose Beneyto is a Chinese martial arts instructor, specializing in Choy Lee fut Kungfu and Lohan Chikung. He has had the opportunity to learn both disciplines from some of the best masters that exist today.

He has also studied in depth the basic theories of traditional Chinese medicine, as well as various oriental techniques for health care, such as acupuncture, Tui na massage or phytotherapy among others.

www.josebeneyto.com

www.luohanqigong.com

https://www.instagram.com/jose.beneyto/

https://www.facebook.com/lohanqigong/

lohanchikung@yahoo.es

AUTHOR'S NOTE

Throughout this book some words from the Chinese language are used. I have used pinyin, which is a phonetic transcription system of Mandarin Chinese and is officially recognized in the People's Republic of China. It changes the use of traditional Chinese characters from conceptual to phonetic. That is, the Latin script is used to phonetically transcribe the Chinese language.

The pinyin system has a complex system of diacritics to mark the tones. In other words, a series of accents and hyphens are used to indicate how the pronunciation should be. None of these signs should be omitted for correct writing.

But throughout the book some words are repeated very much and in order to facilitate its reading I decided to eliminate these diacritics. In order not to lose rigor and for information purposes, I enclose the correct way to write the most used Chinese terms in this book in pinyin. Anyway, you can see that the first time each of them appears in the book, they are written correctly.

Pinyin	Forms Used In The Book
Yīn	Yin
Yáng	Yang
Sānbǎo	Sanbao
Jīng	Jing
Qì	Qi
Shén	Shen
Qìgōng	Qigong
Dāntián	Dantian

Printed in Germany
by Amazon Distribution
GmbH, Leipzig

18356007R00048